Easy Diet:

30 Delicious And Healthy Smoothies for Fast Weight Loss

Table of Contents

Introduction

I would first like to thank and congratulate you for downloading my book **"Smoothies Diet: 30 Delicious, Mouthwatering Smoothies for Easy Weight Loss!"** By adding these wonderful smoothie recipes to your diet and making sure to drink lots of water every day you will be amazed at how better you are going to look and feel.

The average person should consume at least eight glasses of water a day more if you are doing active physical activities or are sweating a lot. You have to make sure that you keep drinking lots of water as this will help your body to function in a much healthier fashion and help cleanse your system keeping you hydrated.

If you want to lose weight and eat healthier choices then a smoothie is a great choice that is packed with healthy ingredients that can help you to reach your weight loss goal while also drinking lots of water as well this combination will help you lose weight in a healthy way.

The great news with this is that you do not have to be on any specific diet plan but adding smoothies into your daily meal plans in place of a meal will make a big difference in your health in a positive way. Train yourself to drink lots of water instead of drinking sodas or other sugar-filled drinks. The best and healthiest drink that you can choose is water, it will help you to stay hydrated and lose weight.

Chapter 1. I Fell in Love with Smoothies!

I started making smoothies about six years ago and I have loved them since day one. I myself try to make at least three smoothies for myself during the week for breakfast. I find the days that I am taking healthy smoothies they are having a positive impact on my overall health. I feel much more energized when I have had a smoothie for breakfast compared to having a couple of cups of coffee and no breakfast.

My old eating habits were nothing to brag about, but when I began to add smoothies into my diet things starting looking up for me in the health department. I felt that my fitness, energy levels, and even my skin was looking better.

Adding smoothies and drinking more water each day really made a great difference in how I was feeling and looking. My skin used to be so dry and wrinkled it was awful. When I began to drink water, lots of water each day and drink smoothies this super combo was making me look and feel better than I had in many years.

I love to experiment with my smoothies I will mix a few things together and then do the taste test to see how my new recipe turned out. I have to admit some of them were not that great but the majority of them where great! I do not want to make the same kind of smoothie over and over I love to try new and different things and that includes trying new flavours of smoothies.

I would find it would be too boring having the same smoothie over and over I like to spice things up in life and that includes adding new smoothies to my diet. Sometimes I will make one big jug full that will last me for a few smoothies.

It is great doing this especially on busy week days when I am rushing around from home to work and back again. I sometimes will even freeze portions of my smoothies to use them at another time.

Smoothies are such a wonderful beverage that are just packed with amazing energy boosting ingredients that will make you feel so energized and ready to take on the challenges of the day.

I find that when I drink smoothies in the morning they give me that extra jump start that I need to get myself up and running giving my a great burst of energy. I am energized for about four hours straight after I have had a breakfast smoothie. I have to keep healthy and motivated so that I can work a full day and come home and spend time with my loved ones.

I feel that I have much more energy on the days that I start them with a smoothie. Days when I do not have my smoothies I feel like I am dragging my feet and lacking energy. Smoothies are loved by all ages, they are a fun yummy healthy drink that you will not have to force your kids to drink—they will want a smoothie because they simply taste yummy! It is certainly an easy way to get your kids to eat their fruits and veggies.

Health Benefits of Smoothies. Smoothies offer many health benefits that will help to keep your body functioning in a healthy manner. It is important that we try to maintain a healthy balance of minerals and vitamins with regular smoothie consumption this can help achieve this.

Consuming too much saturated fat, or taking too much of one vitamin is not good either. Balance of all the healthy minerals that we need to stay healthy is important. The best way for us to achieve this balance is to eat a healthy portion of fruits and veggies daily.

Weight loss. Adding smoothies to your diet is a great way to help you to lose weight. Just by taking a daily smoothie you can lose weight. Many people have lost weight when they began adding smoothies to their daily diets. Along with the smoothies it is a great idea to make your choice of drink good old water.

The more water you drink the better you will feel. You will be able to eat other foods with smoothies and you are still going to see that you have lost weight in a months time. If you are zeroing in on just loosing weight then you should make smoothies that include in them low carb ingredients.

Energy. You will gain enough energy from a breakfast smoothie to last you right up until lunch time. This is one of the best and healthiest choices for breakfast. If you make a leafy green smoothie you will not need to consume anything for another six hours.

Detoxifying Qualities. Drinking a lot of water will help to detoxify your body but so can drinking a smoothies also can have a detoxifying effect on your body. They can help with making your entire system purified while allowing your digestion to improve. If you or someone you love is suffering from constipation or indigestion you should try drinking smoothies as these can be a great alternative to artificial medicines for these health conditions.

Skin improvement. Many people that have added smoothies to their daily diets have noticed that their skin has improved looking much clearer and smoother. They have found their complexion looks so much healthier than it did before they introduced smoothies into their diets.

Often with busy lifestyles people struggle to get the vitamins and nutrients that they need to stay healthy, drinking smoothies can be a great and tasty way to get the nutrients that you need in order to maintain good health and skin.

Can help reduce food cravings. When you add smoothies to your diet you will find that they will help reduce food cravings as they are going to make you feel fuller and more energized than you have in a long time.

You will not feel the urge or the need to binge eat before meals. Often when we feel hungry between meals we will often turn to junk foods that are packed with sugars to temporarily reduce our hunger. You can avoid these unhealthy food choices by simply adding a smoothie to your daily diet.

A few tips for making smoothies. When it comes to making smoothies the great thing about them is there is not hard set way to make them or set ingredients for them. You do not have to stress if you do not have all the ingredients for a smoothie recipe, instead you can get creative and add new ingredients coming up with your own special smoothie.

You have to keep in mind that the fruits and veggies that you use in your smoothie will certainly affect the colour it will end up being. If you are looking to make a red smoothie then using kale and spinach will not give you that red colour you are seeking. You can adapt the ingredients in your smoothies to suit your own personal tastes. Don't be afraid to add new fruits and veggies to your smoothies!

The recipes in this book have been developed to help ensure that the ingredients in them will help give you the health benefits you are seeking.

If you are adding smoothies to your diet because you want to lose weight, then you should avoid adding artificial sweeteners to your smoothies. Avoid adding empty calories into your smoothies.

When you are adding dairy products into your smoothies make sure that they are compatible with the ingredients that you are choosing. If you do not want to use dairy milk you can also use almond, coconut or cashew nut milk as these will work well in a smoothie.

You may even want to add spices into your smoothie to add to the flavor and taste. Adding spices such as cardamom and cinnamon work well in smoothies. Herbs such as mint and coriander leaves are nice to add to your smoothies as well. When making veggie smoothies you might want to try adding garlic or ginger into them to add to the flavour as well as health benefits.

I often add coconut water to my smoothies when they are too thick this is a healthy choice to help thin your smoothies out.

What type of equipment you will need to make smoothies. The equipment you will need to begin making yourself healthy smoothies are a blender, knife, chopping board and a nice tall glass to enjoy your smoothie in! I myself use a NUTRiBULLET blender for my smoothies it works great and has my smoothie made up in no time. There are an assortment of different versions of this blender I am sure that you will have no problem finding the one that is right for you.

I have the original version of NUTRiBULLET it is 600 watts with 20,00 RPM and 511/680ml Capacity. This version is good for making single smoothies. The larger versions are more powerful and larger to make more than one at a time.   If you look online under NUTRiBULLET you will see the different versions available to you.

Creating your own smoothie recipes! The great thing about making smoothies is that you can explore and try adding new fruits and veggie combinations to make your own signature smoothies. Adding many things together such as mint, honey, banana, yogurt and coconut water just to name a few. Have a wonderful time creating new flavours with your smoothies.

You can use the recipes in this book as base recipes adding in different extra ingredients to make them work for your own personal taste. I hope that you will enjoy trying and adding the smoothie recipes in this book to your daily diet. This collection of recipes can certainly help to make your weight loss process a much faster and healthier process along with a healthy lifestyle. You can benefit from them also because of their anti-aging properties, detoxifying your body while they taste great on top of it all!

Chapter 2. Yummy Super Food Smoothies Recipes

1. Pineapple-Orange Smoothie

Servings: 2-3

Ingredients:

- one cup of pineapple, diced
- one orange, peeled
- five dates, deseeded
- four ice cubes
- half a cup of pineapple juice
- one papaya, deseeded
- coconut water as needed

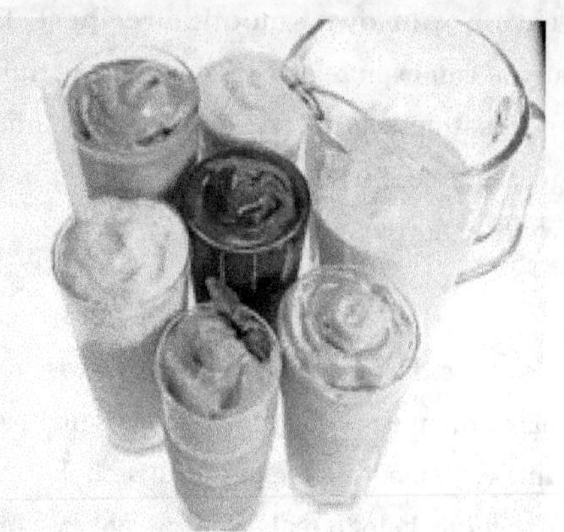

Directions:

Take your dates, papaya, and orange and deseed them. Cut your pineapple into small chunks. Add all of your ingredients into your blender and blend until smooth pour and enjoy!

Health Benefits:

The nutrients of vitamin C, beta-sisterol (this helps to prevent the growth of tumours), fiber, along with digestive enzymes (such as bromelain and papain) manganese and copper.

2. Cashew &Kiwi Smoothie

Serves: 1-2

Ingredients:

- one kiwi fruit

- two tablespoons of organic honey

- one cup of fruit yogurt

- five hazelnuts

- ten cashew nuts

- one quarter of a cup of cranberries, frozen

Directions:

First peel kiwi fruit cut into pieces, add kiwi, nuts, yogurt, honey, cranberries into blender. Blend well if it is too thick add in some water to thin smoothie.

Health Benefits:

You will gain a good source of dietary fiber from this smoothie recipe along with vitamins E and Bs, magnesium, antioxidants, potassium, and proanthocyanidin.

This smoothie recipe can help with preventing urinary tract infections, will cease microbrial growth at infected areas within your body, and will help in maintaining endothelial cell functioning, will decrease LDL cholesterol improving blood quality, also aids in keeping your nervous system in order, the high potassium levels in this smoothie recipe helps reduce blood pressure, and helps maintain electrolyte balance in your body.

3. Anti-oxidant Smoothie

Servings: 1-2

Ingredients:

- half a cup of strawberries, fresh or frozen, chopped

- half a cup of sparkling mineral water

- one teaspoon of Acai powder

- one cup of coconut water

- one tablespoon of almond butter

- a dash of cinnamon powder

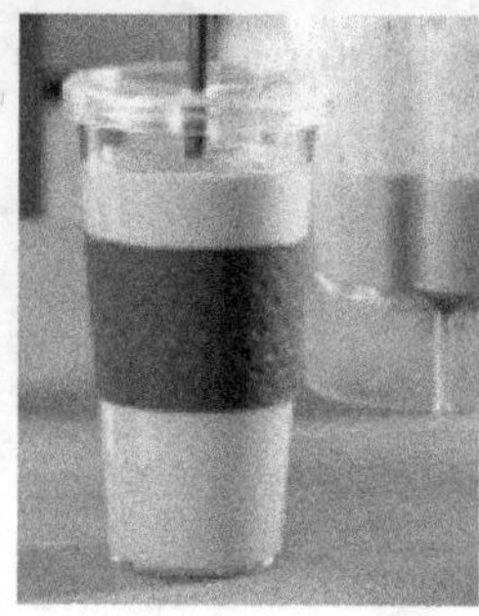

Directions:

Chop and clean your strawberries. Add all the ingredients for smoothie into your blender except for the mineral water. Blend until it is nice and smooth. Add in the mineral water and blend again. Pour smoothie into a glass and top with a dash of cinnamon.

Health Benefits:

This smoothie is an isotonic drink, it has the same osmotic pressure that your body fluids have. This is a great anti-aging smoothie that contains vitamins, A, E, and C as well as antioxidants, magnesium and other nutrients that have super health benefits.

This is a fast-working antioxidant that will scavenge for free-radicals and will neutralize any that may have a potentially negative effect that could damage your cells, it will also help promote eye health, boost your immunity, fight cancer, will increase the production of collagen, will fight bad cholesterol, will boost your heart health and is an anti-inflammatory.

4. Berry & Kefir Smoothie

Servings: 1-2

Ingredients:

- two tablespoons of flaxseeds, whole
- half a cup of kefir
- one cup of blackberries
- two ice cubes
- water as needed

Directions:

Put all of your smoothie ingredients into your blender and blend until smooth, adding water as needed to thin out smoothie as you like it.

Health Benefits:

This is a smoothie that is vitamin packed, calcium-rich, and filled with fiber. The flax seed adds fiber, omega 3 fatty acids and antioxidants, giving your smoothie a little bit of a crunch to it.

5. Coconut & Pomegranate Smoothie

Servings: 1-2

Ingredients:

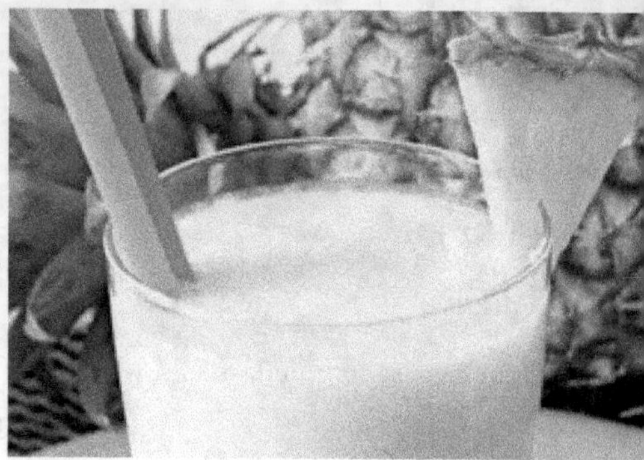

- half a cup of light coconut milk
- one cup of pomegranate seeds
- half a cup of spinach leaves, chopped
- one tablespoon of Chia seeds
- half a cup of kale, chopped
- three ice cubes

Directions:

Add all of your smoothie ingredients to the blender and blend then enjoy your smoothie!

Health Benefits:

This smoothie recipe is full of antioxidants, especially the powerful polyphenols that are thought to help with heart health as well as anti-cancer benefits.

6. Chocolate Blueberry Smoothie

Servings: 1

Ingredients:

- half a cup of blueberries, fresh

- one tablespoon of cocoa powder

- one quarter of a teaspoon of Vanilla extract

- one cup of almond milk, pure, original

Directions:

Add all of your smoothie ingredients into your blender and blend until they are smooth.
Now enjoy your nice fresh chocolate blueberry smoothie.

Health Benefits: This smoothie is great for the nervous system and heart health, as
well as helping with stabilizing your mood. It is also has antioxidants.

7. Mixed Berries Smoothie

Servings: 2

Ingredients:

- one cup of strawberries, chopped

- one cup of blueberries, fresh

- one tablespoon of lemon juice

- one cup of mint tea, unsweetened, chilled

- one tablespoon of Chia seeds

- one cup of coconut water

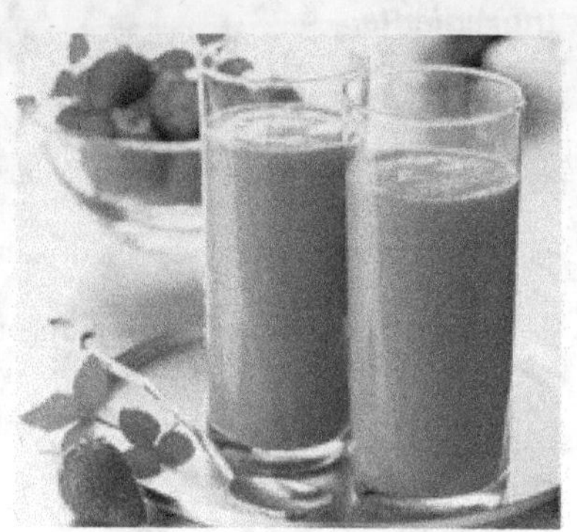

Directions:

Add all of your smoothie ingredients to blender and blend until smooth then enjoy this yummy glass full of healthy!

Health Benefits:

This smoothie is a great source of vitamin C. Vitamin C is great with helping cell growth to occur and can help to reduce wrinkles, remove circles from eyes and make skin texture better. The vitamin C will also aid with regenerating other vitamins in your body such as vitamin E.

8. Summer Watermelon Smoothie

Servings: *4*

Ingredients:

- two lemons, organic with skin

- six cups of watermelon, seedless, cubed

- low-fat vanilla yogurt

- eight ice cubes

Directions:

Put all of your smoothie ingredients into your blender and blend until smooth. This is a wonderful smoothie to enjoy on a hot summer day!

Health Benefits:

This yummy smoothie will help refresh your mood with anti-cancer, anti-aging properties filled with nutrients and low in calories. This is a smoothie that has zero fat content that will be a great smoothie for those trying to manage their weight.

9. Avocado & Mango Smoothie

Servings: 1

Ingredients:

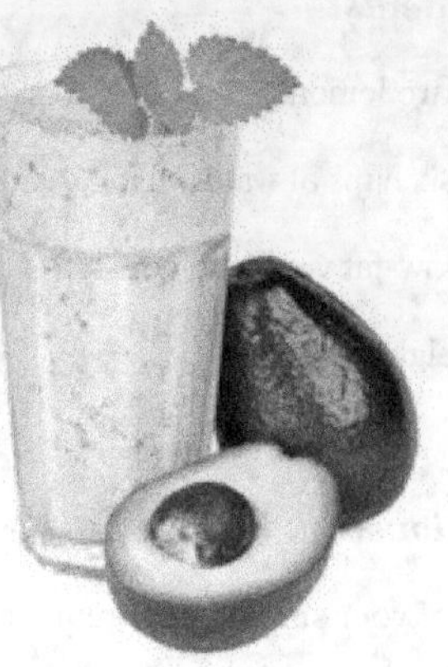

- one quarter of a cup of avocado, ripe, mashed, with outer skin and seed removed

- one quarter cup of mango, skin and seed removed, chunks

- half a cup of mango juice

- one tablespoon of lime juice

- one quarter of a cup of vanilla yogurt, fat-free

- six ice cubes

Directions:

Add all of your smoothie ingredients into blender and blend until smooth and enjoy!

Health Benefits:

This smoothie offers you anti-cancer properties, will help improve your digestion, promote cell health and weight loss.

10. Peach & Banana Smoothie

Servings: 1-2

Ingredients:

- one cup of peach slices, frozen

- one cup of banana, slices, frozen

- one quarter of a cup of blueberries, frozen

- half a cup of vanilla yogurt, fat-free

- cold water as needed

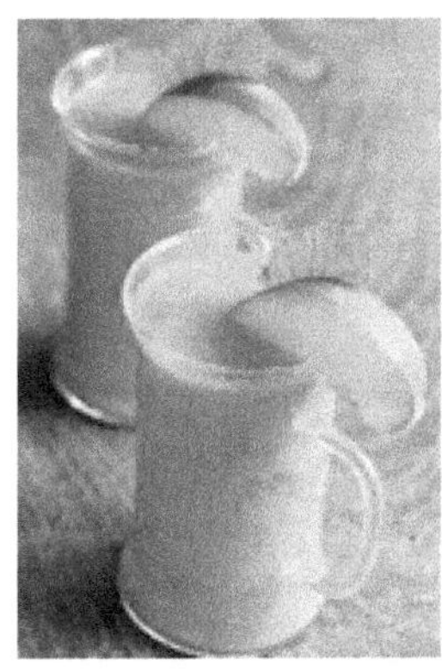

Directions:

Add all of your smoothie ingredients into blender and blend until smooth and enjoy!

Health Benefits:

This great smoothie can provide protection against free-radicals that have negative impacts on your body being that it is high in antioxidants. This smoothie recipe will help avoid cardiovascular diseases, maintain blood cholesterol levels and will also contribute to weight-loss.

11. Coriander & Mint Smoothie

Servings: 2

Ingredients:

- one bunch of coriander, fresh, with stalks

- twelve mint leaves

- half a cup of green tea, brewed, chilled

- half a cup of almond milk, non-fat

- eight ice cubes

Directions:

Put all of your ingredients into blender and blend 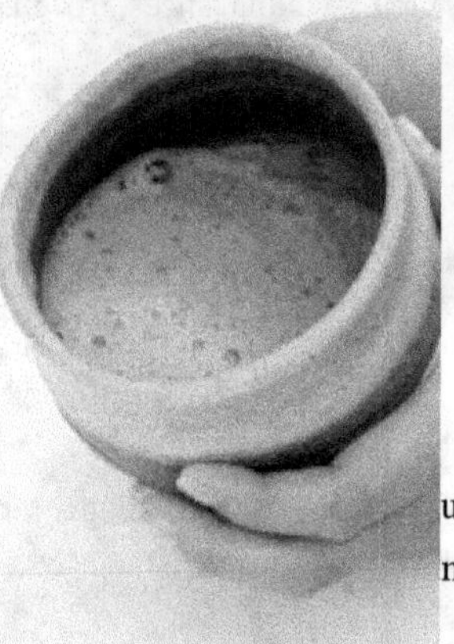 until smooth except tea. Brew tea and chill then add to mixture and blend again.

Health Benefits:

The green tea in the smoothie offers weight-loss benefits due to the Epigallocatechin Gallate (EGCG) that it contains, this substance can boost metabolism and is a health-boosting antioxidant.

This is a lactose-free smoothie that is very rich in Vitamins, C and K. It also contains small amounts of potassium, phosphorous, thiamin, niacin, carotene and calcium. Other benefits provided by this smoothie recipe are relieve of depression, digestion problems, fatigue, respiratory problems, and skin related issues.

12. Yummy Fruit Cocktail Smoothie

Servings: 2

Ingredients:

- one orange peeled

- one apple, cored and sliced

- half a cup of pineapple, cubed

- two and a half cups of watermelon, cubed and seeded

- a sprig of fresh mint

- one teaspoon of lemon juice

Directions:

Juice the apple, orange and pineapple. Transfer to your blender add in the watermelon, lemon juice and mint then blend until smooth and enjoy!

Health Benefits:

This smoothie recipe is filled with antioxidants, high in fiber, phytonutrients, vitamins and minerals. It will also help improve your circulation, heart health and skin.

13. Lavender & Mulberry Smoothie

Servings: 1

Ingredients:

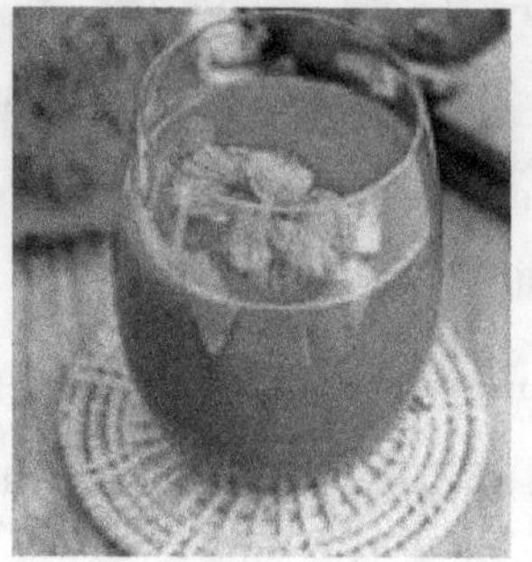

- one cup of mulberries, fresh

- one banana, sliced, frozen

- one tablespoon of lavender, dried

- one cup of apple juice

- half a cup of rolled oats, organic

- 20 cashews, raw

- one teaspoon of vanilla extract

Directions:

Blend all of your smoothie ingredients then top drink with crushed cashews.

Health Benefits:

This smoothie recipe is a great source for antioxidants, vitamins, phytonutrients, giving you immune support, reducing your risk of developing cancer, hypertension, heart disease or diabetes and is good protection for your brain.

14. Tasty Hazlenut-Coffee Smoothie

Servings: 1-2

Ingredients:

- half a cup of coffee, iced

- one quarter of a cup of hazelnuts

- one banana, sliced, frozen

- half a cup of plain Greek yogurt, non-fat

- one teaspoon of vanilla extract

Directions:

Mix all ingredients in a cup except for the coffee. Add ingredients into your blender including coffee and blend until smooth.

Health Benefits:

Great for helping to improve brain functioning, keeping your heart healthy and giving your metabolism is a boost.

15. Apple & Date Smoothie

Servings: 1-2

Ingredients:

- two apples, cored, sliced

- two dates, pitted

- one banana, sliced, frozen

- three tablespoons of hemp protein

- one cup of almond milk

- one quarter of a cup of cashews, raw

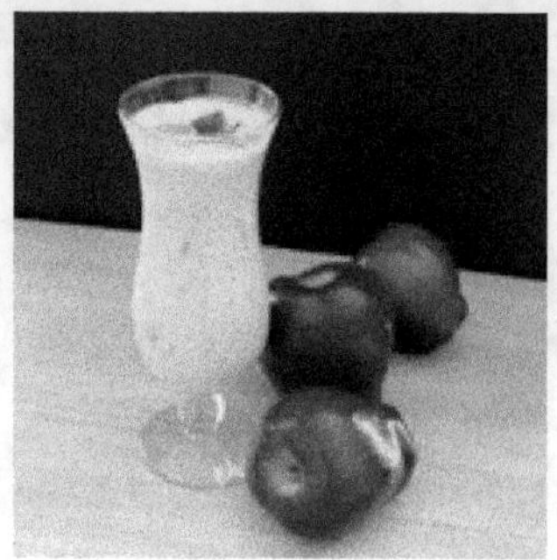

Directions:

Blend all of your smoothie ingredients in blender until nice and smooth. Perhaps sprinkle top of smoothie with cinnamon or apple pie spice.

Health Benefits:

This smoothie recipe is a great energy booster and is good for skin health.

16. Melon Grapefruit Smoothie

Servings: 4

Ingredients:

- one cup of fresh grapefruit juice

- four cups of watermelon, cubed and seeded

- ten ice cubes

- 4 sprigs of mint

Directions:

Add all of your smoothie ingredients, except sprigs of mint, into your blender and blend until smooth. Pour mix into serving glasses and top each glass with a sprig of mint.

Health Benefits:

This smoothie recipe offers anti-inflammatory, and anti-cancer benefits as well as improving your brain health and breath.

17. Berries & Pineapple Smoothie

Servings: 2

Ingredients:

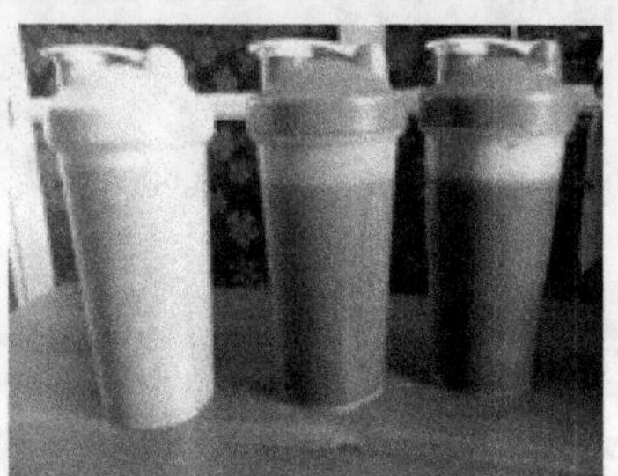

- one cup of strawberries, frozen, sliced

- one cup of pineapple, chunks, fresh

- one cup of pure orange juice

- one mango, ripe, peeled, seeded, diced

- eight ice cubes

Directions:

Add all of your smoothie ingredients to blender and blend until smooth, add ice and serve.

Health Benefits:

This smoothie recipe has anti-cancer benefits and is an energy booster as well as being very rich in nutrients.

18. Melon Smoothie

Servings: 2

Ingredients:

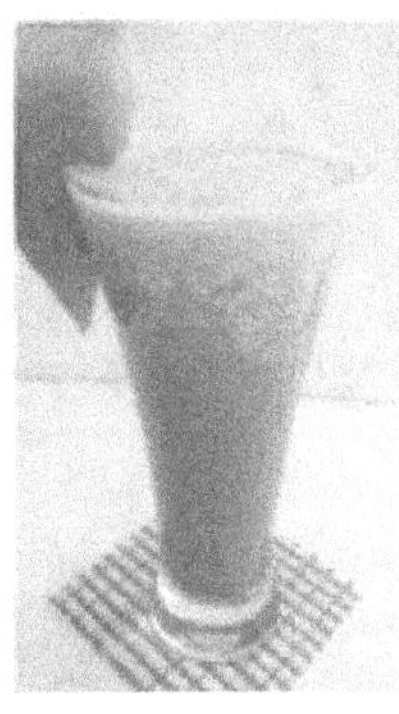

- one cup of cantaloupe, cubed, deseeded

- one cup of watermelon, seeds removed, cubed

- one cup of strawberry juice, use for smoothie base

- half a cup of honeydew melon, chunks

Directions:

Put all of your smoothie ingredients into blender and blend until smooth and enjoy!

Health Benefits:

This smoothie recipe offers antioxidants that will help with treating blood pressure issues and heart diseases. It also has anti-cancer and anti-inflammatory benefits.

19. Fruit & Cucumber Smoothie

Servings: 1

Ingredients:

- one stalk of celery, fresh, chopped

- half a cucumber, peeled and sliced

- a handful of kale, fresh, chopped

- one pear, peeled, sliced

- one apple, peeled, sliced, cored

- one teaspoon of lemon juice

- water as needed

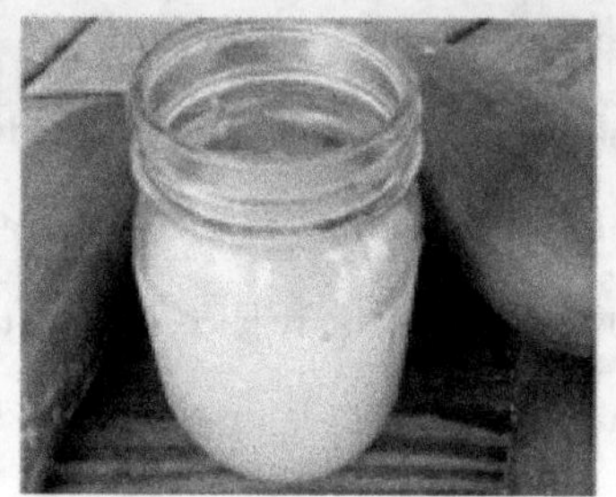

Directions:

Put all of your smoothie ingredients into blender and blend until smooth and enjoy!

Health Benefits:

This smoothie recipe offers you a lot of antioxidants, vitamins, nutrients, dietary fiber, and is also a great source of iron that can help to reduce risks of you contracting a urinary infection.

It is good at helping in preventing cancer, improves the function of the immune functions, decreases blood pressure and also help in lowering the risk of developing cardiovascular diseases.

20. Tangerine Strawberry Smoothie

Servings: 1

Ingredients:

* half a cup of strawberries, frozen, sliced

* one red grapefruit, juiced

* one cup of Tangerine juice, use as base for smoothie

* ice as needed

Directions:

Peel and juice your tangerines then add all of your ingredients into your blender and blend until smooth then enjoy!

Health Benefits:

This smoothie recipe will help with eye to heart health and is jam packed with vitamin C.

21. Berries & Chocolate Smoothie

Servings: 2

Ingredients:

* half a cup of soy milk

* one cup of raspberries, frozen, chopped

* one cup of strawberries, frozen, sliced

* one quarter of a cup of chocolate chips

* half a cup of vanilla yogurt, fat-free

* add water if needed

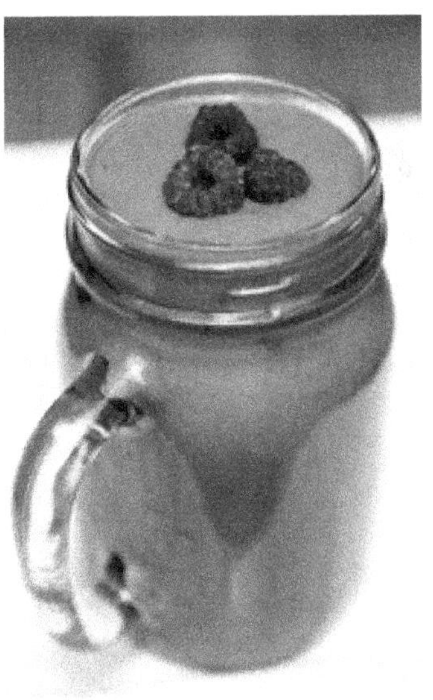

Directions:

Put all of your smoothie ingredients into blender and blend until smooth and enjoy!

Health Benefits:

This smoothie recipe is rich in vitamin C and has less fat content, it contains components of quercetin and gallic acid that help in treating heart diseases, age-related cell decline, and cancer. It contains anti-inflammatory properties and is high in ellagic-acid, known to be a chemopreventative due to the raspberries in the smoothie.

22. Kiwi Cantaloupe Smoothie

Servings: 3

Ingredients:

- two cups of cantaloupe, seeds removed, cubed
- one Kiwi fruit, peeled, chopped
- one tablespoon of lemon juice
- one apple, cored, chopped
- one cup of ice cubes
- water as needed

Directions:

Put all of your smoothie ingredients into blender and blend until smooth and enjoy!

Health Benefits:

This smoothie recipe is a good source of dietary fiber; that will be a great source of potassium, help improve digestion, will help maintain blood homoeostasis, balance blood pressure and water-electrolytes, is also a good source of Vitamin C and copper. These will help to improve your skin by helping with the production of collagen and the repair of skin tissue.

23. Banana, Orange Smoothie

Servings: 2

Ingredients:

- half a cup of vanilla yogurt fat-free

- one cup of strawberries, fresh, sliced

- one banana, ripe, fresh, chopped

- half an orange, sliced

- six ice cubes

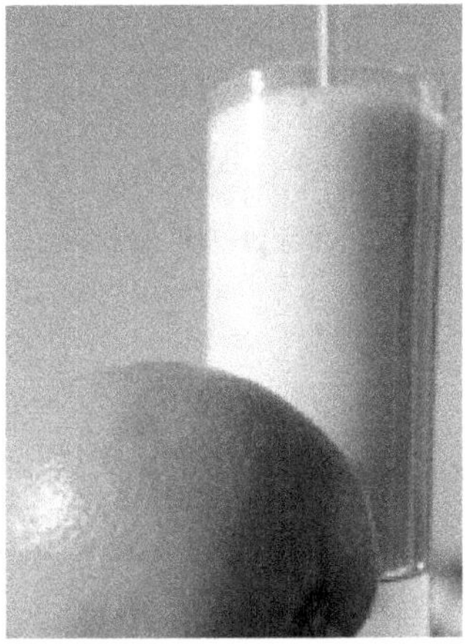

Directions:

Add all of your smoothie ingredients to blender and blend until smooth and enjoy!

Health Benefits:

This smoothie recipe is full of nutrients, and antioxidants, it contains almost no fats, it prevents the storage of belly fats and as a result you will lose weight.

24. Chocolate & Egg Smoothie

Servings: 2

Ingredients:

- half a cup of banana, frozen, sliced

- one quarter of a cup of raspberries, fresh

- four teaspoons of cocoa powder

- two cups of spinach, chopped

- one egg

- one cup of vanilla soy milk

- one tablespoon of flax meal

- one teaspoon of protein powder

- six ice cubes

Directions:

Add all of your ingredients to your blender and blend until smooth then enjoy!

Health Benefits:

This smoothie recipe is very rich in vitamins, protein, minerals, antioxidants, that will help to improve the health of your heart, brain, and skin health. This smoothie has zero cholesterol it makes a great diet drink as it will relieve the satiety hormones in your brain.

25. Blueberries & Oatmeal Smoothie

Servings: 2

Ingredients:

- half a cup of oats, rolled, whole grains

- half a cup of blueberries

- three tablespoons of organic honey

- one cup of milk, low-fat

- one third of a cup of vanilla Greek yogurt

- half a cup of ice

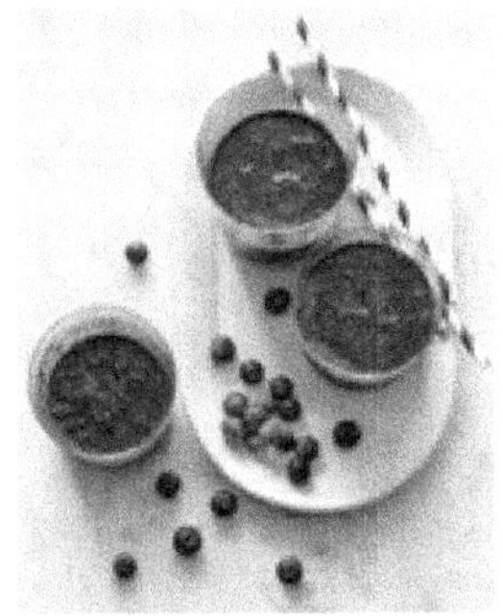

Directions:

Add all of your smoothie ingredients to your blender and blend until smooth then enjoy!

Health Benefits:

This smoothie recipe will help in reducing the risk of cardiovascular diseases. It is also a great source of antioxidants, B vitamins, magnesium, and iron. This smoothie can also help in fighting oxidative stress that is caused by free radicals that can lead to serious illness.

26. Carrot & Walnut Smoothie

Servings: 2

Ingredients:

- one carrot, large, peeled, and chopped

- four walnut kernels

- one cup of cherries, frozen

- six ice cubes

- water as needed

Directions:

Using a grinder grind the walnuts to almost a powder like consistency. Add all of the ingredients into your blender and blend until smooth and enjoy!

Health Benefits:

This smoothie recipe contains antioxidants, will help in improving your cell functions, control cholesterol levels, anti-inflammatory, prevents cancer, will control belly fat and joint pains.

27. Raspberry Coconut Smoothie

Servings: 2

Ingredients:

- one and a half cups of raspberries, frozen

- two cups of coconut milk

- half a teaspoon of vanilla extract

- two egg yolks

- twelve drops of liquid Stevia

- six ice cubes

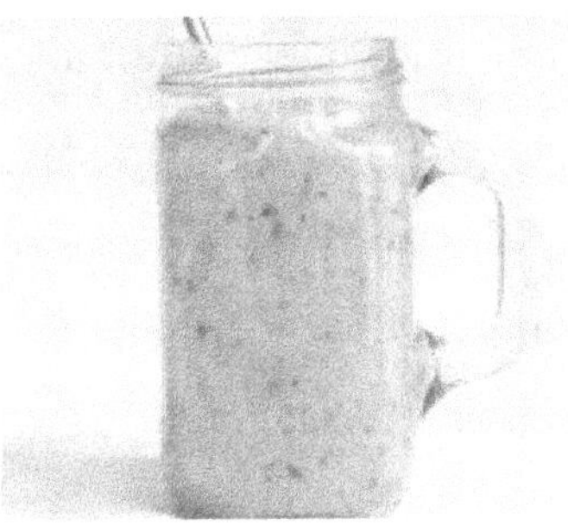

Directions:

Add all of your ingredients into blender except for the walnut powder. Blend until smooth then pour into serving glasses and top with walnut then enjoy!

Health Benefits:

This smoothie recipe is rich in antioxidants, especially ellagic-acid, gallic-acid, quercetin, vitamin C, and minerals that will help to prevent the growth of cancerous cells, will provide the best conditions for cell metabolic processes, will improve blood circulation, skin texture will improve and will decrease the risk of cardiovascular diseases.

28. Milk Thistle & Berries Smoothie

Servings: 2

Ingredients:

- half a cup of blueberries, fresh

- one teaspoon of milk thistle seeds, finely ground or liquid extract

- one banana, frozen, chopped

- one cup of almond milk

- one fig, dried

- half a teaspoon of vanilla extract

- one third of a cup of Goji berries

Directions:

Grind up the milk thistle seeds and soak them in pure water overnight. Put the Goji berries and other ingredients into blender and blend until smooth.

Health Benefits:

This smoothie recipe is great as a liver and blood tonic. It will protect your liver, will cleanse and cause cell regeneration, will help prevent and cure acute liver diseases.

29. Green Tea & Pear Smoothie

Servings: 1

Ingredients:

- half a cup of green tea, brewed, chilled

- one apple, cored, chopped

- one pear, cored, chopped

- one quarter of a cup of mineral water

- pinch of cinnamon

Directions:

Brew your tea then allow it to cool in the refrigerator. Peel and core your apple and pear. Place ingredients into blender except cinnamon. Blend until smooth then pour into serving glass and top with a pinch of cinnamon and enjoy!

Health Benefits:

This smoothie recipe contains phytonutrients and antioxidants, it has great benefits in improving brain function, fights allergies, helps to lower risk of developing cancer, improves the blood circulation, helps to reduce the risk of diabetes and reduces the risk of developing cardiovascular diseases and high blood pressure.

30. Cruciferous Detox Smoothie

Servings: 4-5

Ingredients:

- one cup of cabbage, fresh, chopped

- one cup of broccoli, fresh, chopped

- half a cup of cauliflower, fresh, chopped

- two cups of green tea, brewed, chilled

- half a cup of Brussels sprouts, fresh, chopped

- two tablespoons of organic honey

- two mint leaves

- four ice cubes

- dash of cinnamon

Directions:

Chop up all of the cruciferous veggies put into blender and blend until smooth. Pour into serving glasses with a dash of cinnamon and enjoy!

Conclusion

I hope that you and your loved ones will enjoy and benefit from my collection of smoothie recipes. What I love about smoothies is they are so packed with health benefits and they taste so good it is almost hard to believe that these great tasting drinks are packed with so many healthy ingredients!

I hope you will enjoy and love them as much as I have come to enjoy and love them. I wish you great success in adding this healthy choice of foods into your diet. I assure you that you are going to feel and look better than you have in a very long time just by adding these smoothie recipes into your daily diet plan. Now it is time to get blending up your own super smoothies for you to enjoy!

I want to thank you once again for downloading my book it is very much appreciated. If you have a moment I would love it if you would leave a review of my book on Amazon. Best of luck in adding smoothies into your life! It is something that you will have wished you had done sooner—but as the saying goes "It is better late than never."

FREE Bonus Reminder

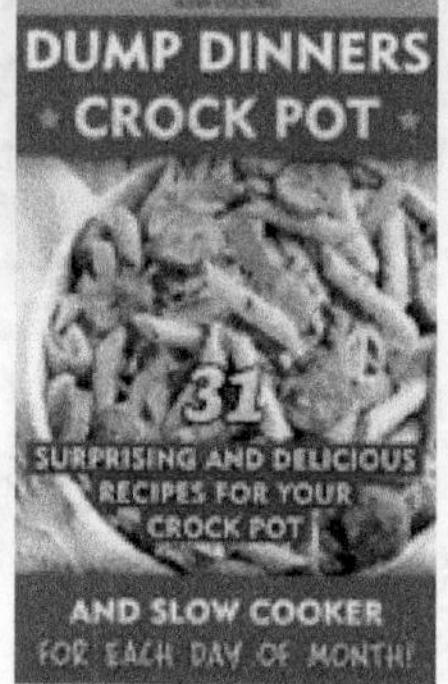

If you have not grabbed it yet, please go ahead and download your Free Ebook
*"Dump Dinners Crock Pot: 31 Surprising And Delicious Recipes For Your Crock
Pot And Slow Cooker For Each Day of Month!"*
Simply Click the Button Below

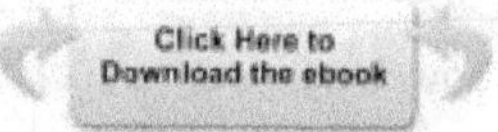

OR **Go to This Page**
http://easycookingideas.com/free

BONUS #2: More Free & Discounted Books

Do you want to receive more Free & Discounted Books?

We have a mailing list where we send out our new Books when they go free or
with a discount on Kindle. Click on the link below to sign up for Free &
Discount Book Promotions.

=> Sign Up for Free & Discount Book Promotions <=

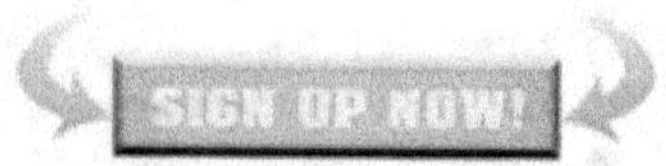

OR Go to this URL
http://zbit.ly/1WBb1Ek

www.ingramcontent.com/pod-product-compliance
Lightning Source LLC
Chambersburg PA
CBHW061741250726
48657CB00002B/1032